The Healthy Eat. To Nourish and Glow Cookbook
(A Beginner's Guide)

Enticing recipes to help get you started on your path to nourishment, happiness and healthy lifestyle.

By Tom Westwood

Copyright © 2015, by: Tom Westwood
All Rights Reserved. No part of this publication may be reproduced in any form or by any means, including scanning, photocopying, or otherwise without prior written permission of the copyright holder.

Disclaimer:
The information provided in this book is designed to provide helpful information on the subjects discussed. The publisher and author are not responsible for any specific health or allergy needs that may require medical supervision and are not liable for any damages or negative consequences from any treatment, action, application or preparation, to any person reading or following the information in this book.

Table of Contents
1. INTRODUCTION
1.1. Eat. Nourish. Glow the 10 easy steps to losing weight, looking younger and feeling healthier
2. The Eat. Nourish. Glow recipes made simple
2.1. Avocado and Mango Salsa
2.2. Bacon Wrapped Chicken Bites
2.3. Asparagus and Swiss cheese Frittata
2.4. Broccoli and Cheese Mini Egg Omelets
2.5. Skinny Coconut Shrimp
2.6. Southwestern Black Bean Salad
2.7. Almond Spice Cookies
2.8. Chicken A La King
2.9. Moo Shu Chicken
2.10. Apple Flax Muffins
2.11. Oven-Baked Salmon with Herbs
2.12. Creamy Spicy Pumpkin Soup
2.13. Flax Meal Pizza Crust
2.14. Cucumber Melon Soup
2.15. Clam Chowder
2.16. Cranberry Vinaigrette
2.17. Artichoke Pesto Dip or Spread
2.18. Bacon, Lettuce, and Tomato Wrap
2.19. Four-Bean Salad
2.20. Egg Nog Recipes
2.21. Vanilla Panna Cotta
2.22. Raspberry Fool
2.23. Raspberry Lemon Mousse
2.24. Raspberry Vanilla Cream
2.25. Strawberry Daiquiri
2.26. Sweet and Sour Lime Dressing
2.27. Spinach Dip
2.28. Coconut Raspberry Muffins
2.29. Cashew cheese recipe
2.30. SPINACH WITH PINE NUTS RECIPE
2.31. HAZELNUT COOKIES RECIPES
2.32. Turkey or Chicken Tetrazzini
2.33. Cauliflower Cheese Soup
2.34. Fajitas - Chicken or Beef
2.35. Fresh Berry Pie
2.36. Lasagna in a Bowl
2.37. Lemon Mousse
2.38. No-Bake Cheesecake
2.39. Peanut Butter Protein Balls
2.40. Pimento Cheese Spread

2.41. Pumpkin Cheesecake
2.42. Sweet and Sour Mix
3. Taco Salad
3.1. Crock Pot Chicken Cacciatore
3.2. Denver Casserole
3.3. Easy Blue Cheese Dressing
3.4. Super-Easy Guacamole
3.5. EASY Chocolate Peanut Butter Fudge
3.6. Easy Shrimp Scampi
3.7. Egg Free Chocolate Mousse
3.8. Five-Minute Sweet Spiced Pecans
3.9. Greek Lemon Garlic Salad Dressing
3.10. Tom Special, Laura Style
3.11. Thai-Style Chicken Salad Recipe
3.12. Old-Fashioned Meat Loaf
3.13. Toasted Pumpkin Seeds
3.14. Seared Scallops
3.15. Strawberry Vinaigrette
3.16. Swordfish Burgers
3.17. Avocado Coconut Popsicles
3.18. Chocolate Ricotta Mousse
3.19. Raspberry Coconut Chia Pudding Pops
3.20. Avocado Egg Salad
3.21. Greek Salad Sandwich
3.22. Cuban sandwich Quesadilla
3.23. Chicken and Andouille Sausage
3.24. CONCLUSION
3.24.1. Thank You

1. INTRODUCTION
Eat. Nourish. Glow the 10 easy steps to losing weight, looking younger and feeling healthier

Amelia Freer brings a fresh and unique voice to the field of holistic health in her bestselling book "Eat. Nourish. Glow.: 10 easy steps for losing weight, looking younger & feeling healthier. In the book she explains her 10 steps and provides over 25 enticing recipes to get you started on your path to nourishment, happiness and healthy lifestyle.

To lose weight is not a shake, a supplement, or an exercise gizmo. The major key to your weight-loss success! **Is right there at your fingertips. I feel the major action you can take when battling to lose weight is to keep a food diary. It is time sapping to write down everything consumed during the day, but this in itself can curtail overeating and be vital for self-assessment and monitoring.**

This book has been written solely with you at heart to guides you gently through her 10 steps, recipes to detox your store cupboards and restock with alternatives. However, this book will guide you on how to understand the differences between good and bad fats, the dangers of hidden sugar in the food we consume and how to dump the wheat from your diet with ideas backed up by the latest findings in the field of nutrition and neuroscience. In addition, you will enjoy all the mouthwatering recipes that will guide you on the path to better health, losing weight and looking great, which has proven not to be easier.

The Eat. Nourish. Glow. Will change your relationship with food, and in turn alter your relationship with yourself and your work. Additionally, it will transform your life and help you lost two stone, dropped two dress sizes and no longer shovel in food like a rabid dog.

2. The Eat. Nourish. Glow recipes made simple

2.1. Avocado and Mango Salsa
Ingredients:
2 avocado (peeled and diced)
2 cloves garlic (minced)
½ cup of chopped fresh cilantro
½ cup of chopped red onion
Salt and fresh pepper
2 mangos (peeled and diced)
2 plum tomatoes (diced)
2 jalepeño (seeded and diced)
4 tablespoons of fresh lime juice
2 tablespoons of olive oil

Directions:
1. First, you combine the entire ingredients and let it marinate in the refrigerator for about 30 minutes before serving.

Nutritional value:
Amount per serving: 1 serving size
Calories: 119.4
Fat: 8.2g
Carbohydrate: 12.6g
Dietary fiber: 3.4g
Protein: 1.3g

2.2. Bacon Wrapped Chicken Bites
Tips:
Meanwhile, you heat oven to a temperature of 375°F.
Ingredients:
20 slices bacon (cut into thirds)
2.50 lbs. (6) boneless skinless chicken breast (cut in 1-inch chunks, about 30 pieces)
Directions:
1. First, you wrap a piece of bacon around each piece of chicken, and then secure with a toothpick and place on a baking sheet (I suggest you use foil for easy cleanup).

2. Then you bake on the lower rack turning halfway approximately 25 minutes, or until thoroughly cooked and browned.

3. After which you blot on a paper towel and serve right away.

Nutritional value:
Amount per serving: 1 serving size
Calories: 70.1
Fat: 2g
Carbohydrate: 0g
Dietary fiber: 0g
Protein: 12.1g

2.3. Asparagus and Swiss cheese Frittata

Ingredients:
1 cup of shallots (chopped)
6 large eggs
2 tablespoons 1% milk
Salt and fresh pepper
1 lb. of asparagus (tough ends trimmed off)
4 teaspoons of butter
10 large eggs whites
4 tablespoons of fresh grated Pecorino Romano
6 oz. reduced fat Swiss cheese (preferably Sargento)

Ingredients:

1. First, you steam asparagus crisp and tender, about 3 to 4 minutes.

2. After which you thinly slice on the diagonal into ½ -inch pieces.

3. Meanwhile, you heat oven to a temperature of 350°F.

4. After that, you heat butter in a 10-inch oven safe skillet over medium heat.

5. At this point, you stir in shallots and sauté for about 4-5 minutes until golden.

6. Then you add steamed asparagus, salt and pepper.

7. Furthermore, you whisk eggs, egg whites, grated cheese, milk, salt, and pepper in a medium bowl.

8. This is when you add the Swiss cheese and mix thoroughly.

9. After which you add eggs to the skillet making sure eggs cover the asparagus.

10. After that, you cook on medium for about 4 minutes, until the edges begin to set.

11. Finally, you move the skillet to oven.

12. Then you cook for about 16 to 18 minutes, or until frittata is completely cooked.

13. Make sure you serve hot, cut into 4 to 6 equal wedges.

Nutritional value:
Amount per serving: 1 serving size
Calories: 226
Fat: 11g
Carbohydrate: 13g
Dietary fiber: 3.5g
Protein: 21g

2.4. Broccoli and Cheese Mini Egg Omelets
Ingredients:
8 whole large eggs
½ cup of reduced fat shredded cheddar (preferably Sargento)
2 teaspoons of olive oil
A cooking spray
8 cups of broccoli florets
2 cups of egg whites
Salt and fresh pepper
½ cup of good grated cheese like pecorino romano
Directions:
1. Meanwhile, you heat oven to a temperature of 350°.

2. After which you team broccoli with a little water for about 6-7 minutes.

3. At a point, when broccoli is cooked, crumble into smaller pieces, you then add olive oil, salt and pepper.

4. After that, you mix thoroughly.

5. Then you spray a standard size of non-stick cupcake tin with cooking spray and spoon broccoli mixture evenly into 9 tins.

6. This is the point when you beat egg whites, eggs, grated cheese, salt and pepper in a medium bowl.

7. Furthermore, you pour into the greased tins over broccoli until a little more than 3/4 full.

8. Finally, you top with grated cheddar and bake in the oven for about 20 minutes until cooked.

9. Make sure you serve immediately.

10. Then you wrap any leftovers in plastic wrap and store in the refrigerator to enjoy later.

Nutritional value:
Amount per serving: 1 serving size
Calories: 167
Fat: 8.5g
Carbohydrate: 5g
Dietary fiber: 2.5g
Protein: 18g

2.5. Skinny Coconut Shrimp
Tips:
Meanwhile, you heat oven to a temperature of 425°.
After which you spray a non-stick baking sheet with cooking spray.
Ingredients:
1cup + 2 tablespoons of shredded sweetened coconut
4 tablespoons of all-purpose flour (you will only use 2 tablespoon)
Non-stick spray (preferably my misto)
2 lb. (48) large raw shrimp, peeled and deveined (make sure you weight after peeled)
1 cup + 2 tablespoons of panko crumbs
2 large eggs
Pinches of salt
Ingredient for the Sweet and Spicy Dipping Sauce:
1 ¼ crushed red pepper flakes
1 cup of apricot preserves (you can use sugar free if you want)
2 tablespoons of rice wine vinegar
Directions:
1. First, you mix together the coconut flakes, panko crumbs and salt in a bowl.

2. After which you put the flour on a small dish and then whisk egg in another bowl.

3. Then you season shrimp with a little salt.

4. At this point, you put the shrimp in the flour, shaking off excess, then into the egg and then into the coconut crumb mixture.

5. Furthermore, you lay shrimp on the cookie sheet then spray the top of the shrimp with more cooking spray.

6. This is when you bake in the middle rack for about 10 minutes.

7. Then you turn shrimp over, and then cook another 6 to 7 minutes or until cooked though.

8. Finally, you remove from oven and serve with dipping sauce.

9. As for the sauce, I suggest you combine the entire ingredients and place in a small bowl.

Nutritional value:
Amount per serving: 1 serving size
Calories: 161.6
Fat: 3.4g
Carbohydrate: 22.2g
Dietary fiber: 1.8g
Protein: 10.2g

2.6. Southwestern Black Bean Salad
Ingredients:
18 oz. of cooked corn, fresh or frozen (preferably thawed if frozen)
2/3 cup of red onion (chopped)
3 - 4 limes, juice of
4 tablespoons of fresh minced cilantro (or more to taste)
2 diced jalapeno (it is optional)
2 (15.5 oz.) cans of black beans (rinsed and drained)
2 medium tomatoes (chopped)
2 scallions (chopped)
2 tablespoons of olive oil
2 medium hass avocado (diced)
Salt and fresh pepper to taste

Directions:
1. First, you combine beans, corn, tomato, onion, scallion, cilantro, salt and pepper in a large bowl.

2. After which you squeeze fresh lime juice to taste and stir in olive oil.

3. Then you marinate in the refrigerator for about 30 minutes.

4. Finally, you add avocado just before serving.

Nutritional value:
Amount per serving: 1 serving size
Calories: 79.5
Fat: 3.5g
Carbohydrate: 12g

Dietary fiber: 3g
Protein: 3g

2.7. Almond Spice Cookies
Ingredients:
1½ Tablespoons of apple pie spice (or 1 teaspoon of cinnamon, ½ teaspoon of nutmeg, and a pinch of cloves)
½ cup of sugar equivalent in artificial sweetener (preferable zero carb, such as liquid sweetener)
½ teaspoon of vanilla
Sliced almonds (it is optional)
2 cups of almond meal (with skins works well)
½ teaspoon of salt
1 packet of artificial sweetener (to sprinkle on top)
1 egg, large

Directions:
1. Meanwhile, you heat oven to a temperature of 325 F.
2. After which you combine all dry ingredients and whisk.
3. Then you add the wet ingredients.
4. Combine very well, until mixture has formed a large ball.
5. Flatten the formed bell with hands or a spoon to about ¼ inch thickness.
6. At this point, you sprinkle powdered sweetener on the tops.
7. After which you place on baking sheet covered with parchment or silicon mat. (Grease the baking sheet alternatively)
8. Then you top with sliced almonds, if you so wished.
9. Finally, you bake for 10 to 12 minutes, or until cookies are slightly brown on bottom.

Nutritional value: each cookie
Amount per serving
Calories: 50
Carb: ½ g
Protein: 2g

Dietary fiber: 1g

2.8. Chicken A La King
Tips:
1. When serving, I suggest you serve over "Cauli-Rice" or low-carb toast (such as the toasted Flax Meal Focaccia Bread) or, any low-carb pasta or pasta substitute works well.

2. I prefer using a half and half approach in preparing this recipe:
3. First, you I use partly a starchy thickener (some type of flour).
4. In the other hand, partly, a low-carb product such as xanthan gum or thicken Thin.

Ingredients:
½ cup of onion, chopped
2 small can of mushrooms (or 4 to 6 oz. fresh chopped mushrooms)
½ teaspoon of black pepper
2 cup of milk or unsweetened soy or almond milk (carb count is for unsweetened soy or almond milk)
2 ½ cups of chicken stock (or water with chicken Better than Bouillon or regular bouillon)
Salt if you not using bouillon
4 cups of cooked chicken or turkey
2 small green pepper, chopped (approximately 3 oz.)
4 Tablespoons of oil or butter
12 Tablespoons of flour (or less flour and a low carb alternative)
1-cup of cream
28 oz. jar of chopped pimentos

Preparation:
1. First, you heat the oil or butter and sauté' the onion for about 2-3 minutes.
2. After which you add the green pepper and mushrooms, and cook until softening.
3. Then you add black pepper.

4. Furthermore, you add the flour, if you using it as a thickener.
5. After which you cook for about 2 minutes before adding liquids.
6. Then you add liquids.
7. At this point, you add the low-carb thickeners, and any flavorings such as better than Bouillon.
8. In addition, you add salt if needed.
9. Then you bring to a simmer and cook for about 3-4 minutes.
10. Finally, you add chicken/turkey and pimento.
11. Then you heat through.

Nutritional value:
Amount per serving
Calories: 237
Carb: 5g
Protein: 17g
Dietary fiber: 1g

2.9. Moo Shu Chicken
TIPS:
1. This recipe has quite a bit of sugar either in it, added directly or in Hoisin sauce, I suggest you use a sugar-free plum sauce.
2. Feel free to substitute packaged Cole slaw mix for the cabbage.
3. However, if you do, do not cook it more than 1 minute or it will become mushy (which is not at all the texture you're going for).

Ingredients:
INGREDIENTS FOR MARINADE:
1 Tablespoon of sesame oil
½ teaspoon of Chinese Five Spice powder
3 Tablespoons of soy sauce
1 clove garlic (crushed)
1 teaspoon of grated fresh ginger
STIR-FRY:
2 medium stalks celery (thinly sliced)
1 Tablespoon of grated fresh ginger
1 cup of sliced green onion (scallions) at approximately 6 onions
1 Tablespoon of soy sauce
1 Tablespoon of oil, you may use vegetable or olive
1 lb. chicken (cut into ½-inch strips)
3 cloves garlic (crushed)
6 oz. of fresh shitake mushrooms (sliced into ½-inch strips)
4 cups of sliced cabbage (approximately ½-inch strips)
8 oz. of bean sprouts (preferably mung beans, or any type intended for stir-frying)

Directions:
1. First, you mix together marinade ingredients, add chicken, and mix to coat.
2. After which you prepare vegetables, and grate ginger and garlic so everything will be ready.
3. After that, you heat large skillet on medium-high heat with olive oil or vegetable.
4. At this point, when the oil is hot, you add the chicken, and stir-fry for about 3 to 4 minutes until just cooked through (depending on how thick you cut the chicken).
5. After which you remove chicken from pan.
6. Then you add the sesame oil, then the celery, ginger, and garlic and sauté for 1 minute.
7. After which you add the vegetables in the order as stated (starting with the mushrooms, onions, cabbage, bean sprouts).
8. Then you stir-frying for about 2 minutes after each addition.
9. Finally, you add the soy sauce and the chicken and then you toss to combine.
10. When serving, I suggest you serve with a sugar-free plum sauce (you can use low-carb tortillas as wrappers, if you choose to).

Nutritional value:
Amount per serving
Calories: 284
Carb: 10g
Protein: 31g
Dietary fiber: 4g

2.10. Apple Flax Muffins
Tips:
1. Meanwhile, you heat oven to a temperature of 350 F.
2. After which you grease a 12-muffin tin very well.

Ingredients:
3 teaspoons of baking powder
1 ½ teaspoon of nutmeg
Artificial sweetener equal to 3/4 cup of sugar (sugar-free syrup can be flavored on 1/2 cup)
¼ cup of oil
1-Tablespoon of vanilla
½ cup of chopped pecans (it is optional)
1 ¼ cup of flax seed meal
1-Tablespoon of cinnamon
½ teaspoon of salt
4 large eggs (beaten)
1 medium apple (chopped fairly finely)
½ cup of liquid (preferable flavored syrup or water)

Directions:
1. First, you mix the dry ingredients together.
2. After which you add the rest of them.
3. Then you let batter stand 10 minutes.
4. After which you then put into the muffin pan and bake for approximately 18 minutes (or until toothpick comes out clean and muffins just barely start to pull away from the sides of the tin).

Nutritional value:
Amount per serving
Carb: 2g
Dietary fiber: 5g

2.11. Oven-Baked Salmon with Herbs
Ingredients:
4 - 8 Tablespoon of fresh herbs, chopped (thyme or dill is nice, but anything that works for you is also good)
2 teaspoons of oil (if that, I suggest you just need a very thin film)
2 salmon filet (approximately 1 pound)
1 teaspoon of pepper
1 teaspoon of salt (put a bit more if kosher or if fish is skinned)
Directions:
1. I saw this technique initially on a segment of Jacques Pepin's TV show "Fast Food My Way".
2. In the show, he does his a bit fancier, by removing the skin (Note that it is not necessary, unless you do not want the unsightly skin hanging around your buffet).
3. First, you heat the oven to a temperature of 200 F.
4. After which you chop up the herb, and mix it with the salt and pepper (Note that regular thyme or any herb you like works fine -even parsley).
5. If you prefer using more, that is okay, and sometimes I mix in 1 tablespoon or so of sesame seeds.
6. Then you smear the oil on an ovenproof serving platter, and place the fish on top.
7. Put some salt and pepper on both sides, if the filet is skinned, otherwise just put the fish skin side down and season the top.
8. Finally, you bake for approximately 40 to 45 minutes, until salmon flakes.
9. After which I promise you will not believe how good it is.
10. I suggest you serve it with a sort of homemade tartar sauce mixing mayonnaise, lemon zest and juice, some of the same herb I used on the fish, capers, and a very little quantity of hot sauce.

Nutritional value:
Amount per serving
Calories: 230
Carb: 0g
Protein: 30g

2.12. Creamy Spicy Pumpkin Soup
TIPS:
1. In the creamy spicy pumpkin soup you can easily double, the recipe by using a large (29 oz.) can of pumpkin.
2. If you are going to use fresh pumpkin, I suggest you just put the pumpkin on a baking sheet, slit it to let out the steam.
3. After which you cook in a 350 F oven until soft, approximately 45 to 60 minutes.
4. Then you split, allow cooling, and scoop out the seeds and pulp.
5. Mash, or I recommend you use a blender or food processor until pumpkin puree is smooth.

Ingredients:
1 small onion (sliced)
1 Tablespoon of grated fresh ginger
1 teaspoon of cinnamon
A pinch cayenne pepper
One 15-16 oz. can pumpkin (note it not pumpkin pie filling)
1 to 2 teaspoons of sugar substitute of your choice
1-Tablespoon of oil
2 cloves garlic (chopped or pressed)
1 Tablespoon of coriander (i.e. ground seed)
¼ teaspoon of nutmeg
½ cup of dry white wine
2 cups of chicken or vegetable broth (feel free to use bouillon)
1 cup ½ and ½

Directions:
1. First, you heat oil and sauté onions until soft, in a large pot or saucepan.
2. After which you add garlic and ginger and cook for another 30 seconds.
3. Then you add the spices for another 30 seconds or so (until fragrant, be careful not to let the spices burn).
4. Furthermore, you add wine, and stir for another minute.
5. After which you remove from heat.
6. Then you add the pumpkin and one cup of liquid.
7. In addition, you puree with stick blender, or in blender or food processor.
8. After which when it is smooth, you heat in pot with the rest of the liquid until simmering.
9. Then you taste.
10. Finally, you add a small amount of sweetener, a little hot sauce or a small amount of raw grated ginger if you want more of a kick.
11. At this point you add salt to taste if you so wish and a bit more sweetener (if the flavors seem a little harsh).
12. For good garnishes, I suggest you included pumpkin seeds, bacon bits, or grated Parmesan or sharp cheddar cheese.

Nutritional value: per serving
Amount per serving
Calories: 134
Carb: 9g
Protein: 3g
Dietary fiber: 3.5g

2.13. Flax Meal Pizza Crust
TIPS:
Preheat oven to a temperature of 425 F.
Ingredients
4 teaspoons baking powder
2 teaspoon of oregano
6 Tablespoons of oil
1 Cup of water
3 Cups of flax seed meal
2 teaspoons of salt
6 eggs
Sweetener to equal approximately 2 Tablespoons of sugar
Directions:
1. First, you mix the dry ingredients together.
2. After which you add wet ingredients, and mix thoroughly.
3. Then you Let sit for approximately 5 minutes to thicken.
4. Furthermore, you spread on pan (I suggest you put it on a silicon mat or greased parchment paper).
5. Finally, you bake for about 15-18 minutes until cooked through.
6. After which you add toppings and cook until they are done.

Nutritional value: whole crust
Amount per serving
Healthy Fat: 130g
Carb: 7g

Protein: 47g
Dietary fiber: 52g

2.14. Cucumber Melon Soup
Tips:
1. This recipe contains cucumber, yogurt, honeydew melon, cilantro, and mint.
2. Feel free to use regular yogurt instead of Greek-style, but if you do, I suggest you add a couple of grams of carbohydrate per serving.

Ingredients:
3 cups of honeydew melon (cubed)
A fistful of cilantro (approximately 1 dozen sprigs, including stems)
Salt and pepper (Note: you start with a bit more than a ¼ teaspoon of salt)
2 large seedless cucumber, or 2 medium peeled regular cucumber (this would be equal to approximately 4 cups of sliced or chopped cucumber)
1 ½ cups of Greek-style yogurt
2 fistful of mint (the leaves from approximately 8 sprigs of mint)

Directions:
1. First, you cut the cucumber into large chunks about five or six pieces.
2. After which you put everything into the blender and blend it up.
3. At this point, you taste (Note that it is going to vary a bit according to the sweetness of the melon, the tartness of the yogurt, etc.
4. Furthermore, you add more mint or cilantro or salt, if you so wish.
5. After which you adjust the amounts to your taste.
6. I suggest you serve this soup with a few small mint leaves as a garnish and a sprinkling of sea salt over the top.

Nutritional value: per serving
Amount per serving
Calories: 64
Carb: 7g
Protein: 3g

Dietary fiber: 1.5g

2.15. Clam Chowder
Tips:
1. Note that 2 tablespoons of flour would only add 14 grams of carb to the whole recipe (so it all depends on your own carb tolerance).
2. I prefer the following thickeners such as guar gum, xanthan gum, or others.

Ingredients:
1 medium onion (chopped small)
2 cloves garlic (pressed or minced)
¾ teaspoon of Old Bay Seasoning (if you like your soup a little spicy, I suggest you use 1 teaspoon)
Low-carb thickener or Flour (see note above)
¾ cup of unsweetened soymilk (if you do not like soy, I suggest you use milk, half and half, or water)
3 cups of cauliflower (chopped)
2 tablespoons of minced fresh parsley
3 pieces of thick-sliced bacon
2 medium celery stalks (chopped small)
¼ teaspoon of black pepper (or ½ teaspoon of celery salt and a pinch of cayenne pepper)
¾ cup of heavy cream
1 cup of clam juice
1 teaspoon of dried thyme (or 1 tablespoon of fresh thyme)
Two 6½ oz. cans of chopped clams (or one 10 oz. can whole baby clams)
Directions:
1. First, you chop the bacon into small cubes and cook until crisp.

2. After which you remove the bacon with a slotted spoon.
3. Then you pour off all but a tablespoon of the rendered fat.
4. At this point, you fry the onion and celery until it starts to soften.
5. Furthermore, you add the garlic and spices except the thyme.
6. After which you stir and cook for about a minute.
7. If you want to use flour to thicken, this is the point when you add it.
8. Then you stir for another 1 to 2 minutes (Note: always count one extra gram of carbohydrate per serving for every tablespoon of flour you add).
9. In addition, you add the liquids and stir.
10. After that, you add the low-carb thickener (I prefer to add it slowly by shaking it through a strainer and whisking it in so it does not clump).
11. Then you stop a little before it gets to your satisfaction (Note that it continue to thickening as the mixture continues to heat).
12. Finally, you turn the heat off when the mixture begins to simmer.
13. After which you steam, boil, or microwave the cauliflower just until fork-tender, then you drain.
14. Then you add clams, thyme, cauliflower, bacon, and parsley.
15. You heat again until it simmers.

Nutritional value: per serving
Amount per serving
Calories: 226
Carb: 6g
Protein: 12g
Dietary fiber: 2g

2.16. Cranberry Vinaigrette
Tips:
This recipe is good on a green salad with blue cheese and toasted nuts.
Ingredients:
1 cup of fresh or frozen cranberries
2/3 cup of olive oil
2 Tablespoon of wine or cider vinegar
Add salt, pepper, and sweetener to taste
2 Tablespoon of water
Directions:
1. First, you put all ingredients in the blender and process until smooth.
2. After which you store in refrigerator.
3. Whole recipe has 4 grams of effective carbohydrate and 2 grams of fiber.

2.17. Artichoke Pesto Dip or Spread
Tips:
1. This recipe goes well with cucumber or jacamars slices or any other vegetables to dip in to it or rather as a spread for low-carb crackers.
2. It is wonderful as a stuffing for mushroom caps and then broiled.
3. Use low fat or fat-free cream cheese, if you looking forward for a South Beach Diet, or to reduce calories.

Ingredients:
6 oz. cream cheese at room temperature (2 small packages or 3/4 of a large one)
1 can artichoke hearts (about 13 oz. to 15 oz.) or 1 package frozen artichoke hearts (no breading), about 9 oz., thawed
1 container of fresh pesto sauce, 7 oz. (usually found near the fresh pasta refrigerated section)

Directions:
1. First, you put the entire ingredients in to the food processor and combine or blend with a stick blender.

Nutritional value: whole serving
Amount per serving
Carb: 17g
Protein: 35g
Dietary fiber: 17g

2.18. Bacon, Lettuce, and Tomato Wrap
Tips:
Feel free to add avocado to this BLTA wrap.
Ingredients:
3 slices of bacon (cooked until crisp and crumbled)
Black pepper to taste
3 to 4 large leaves of green lettuce
2 tablespoons of mayonnaise (regular)
½ cup of raw tomatoes (chopped)
Directions:
· First, you mix chopped tomato with crumbled bacon, mayonnaise, and a generous amount of pepper.
· After which you spoon mixture into the middle of the leaves, and wrap in either a burrito or a taco shape.

Nutritional value: whole recipe
Amount per serving
Calories: 362
Carb: 5g
Protein: 7g
Dietary fiber: 2g

2.19. Four-Bean Salad

Tips:
i. This low-carb four bean salad is sugar-free and the beans are less starchy ones.
ii. Feel free to use kidney beans or chickpeas to substitute for the black soybeans or edamame, but make sure not to use canned beans, because they are more glycerin and have less resistant starch than the dry beans when soaked and cooked by you.
iii. If you prefer a three-bean salad, all you do is use 16 oz. of the green beans and eliminate one of the others.

Ingredients:
One cup of fresh or frozen shelled edamame (fresh soybeans)
¼ cup of fresh parsley (chopped)
1 teaspoon of dried herbs (I prefer Greek or Italian mixtures, on the other way round thyme is good but feel free to use whichever works for you).
12 oz. of green beans, fresh or frozen (preferable canned)
1/3 cup of red Bell pepper (chopped)
3 tablespoons of red wine vinegar
½ teaspoon of garlic powder
One 15 oz. of can yellow string beans (preferable frozen or fresh)
1/3 cup of green Bell pepper (chopped)
1 teaspoon of prepared mustard
½ cup of light olive oil or other oil (see introductory note)
Add salt and pepper to taste
¼ cup of red onion (chopped)
One 15 oz. of can black soybeans

Directions:
1. First, you combine the beans, peppers, onion, and parsley in a large bowl.
2. After, which you mix the vinegar with the mustard and seasonings, either in a small bowl, or a shaker such as a glass jar.
3. Then you add the oil, and whisk or shake to combine.
4. Furthermore, you pour over the beans and vegetables, and toss.

Note on oil:
1. The only disadvantage for using extra-virgin olive oil is that it tends to solidify when refrigerated.
2. An alternative for extra-virgin olive oil is a high-mono type of safflower or sunflower oil such as Saffola brand.
3. However, I am not a fan of using other seed oils like the corn oil or soy oil as they are so high in omega-6 fats.

Nutritional value: per serving
Amount per serving
Calories: 144
Carb: 3g
Protein: 5g
Dietary fiber: 4g

2.20. Egg Nog Recipes

Tips:
1. This Eggnog recipe is traditionally made with raw eggs, milk, sugar, and brandy and/or bourbon and/or rum.
2. If you cherish alcohol, I suggest you add more (I think it tastes great without alcohol at all).

Ingredients:
8 cups i.e. 2 quart of milk (preferable unsweetened soymilk, or unsweetened almond milk)
1 cup of sugar substitute, or more to taste (preferable liquid)
12 eggs
4 cups of heavy cream
½ cup of brandy
Nutmeg
½ cup of rum or bourbon

Directions:
1. Traditionally, eggnog are discouraged nowadays but you have the following alternatives:
2. You should buy pasteurized eggs, if you can find them around.
3. After which you use the recipe to make stirred custard.
4. Then you use half the liquid and add the rest of the liquid after the mixture cools.
5. I suggest you throw caution to the winds and use raw egg, I suggest you use fresh from a farm with a small flock of hens.
6. In addition, you make fake eggnog by substituting Da Vinci's Sugar-Free Egg Nog Syrup for the egg and sweetener.

Two no-cook directions:
Easy Preparatory Directions:
1. First, you put the entire ingredients into a blender and blend it up.
2. After which you sprinkle with nutmeg

The Traditional Preparatory directions:
1. First, you separate the eggs, beat the yolks until light, and the whites until they form soft peaks.
2. You can even whip the cream as well if you so wish.
3. Finally, you combine everything with a whisk (do not over mix).
4. After which you sprinkle nutmeg on the top

2.21. Vanilla Panna Cotta
Tips:
1. Panna cotta is a nice dessert that you can flavor in many ways, such as with berries or a berry sauce.
2. However, you can make it in ramekins or custard cups and unmold it on the plate or bowl.
3. On the other hand, you can pour it into wine glasses or other smallish glasses and serve it right in the glass.

Ingredients:
3 teaspoons of unsweetened gelatin powder
2 pint (4 cups) of heavy cream
A pinch salt to taste
½ cup of cold water
½ cup of boiling water
4 teaspoons of vanilla extract
Sugar substitute (equal to ½ cup sugar)

Directions:
1. First, you sprinkle the gelatin powder on the cold water.
2. After which you let to soften for several minutes.
3. Then you add the boiling water and stir until gelatin is well dissolved (I understand that a fork works well).
4. In addition, you combine dissolved gelatin with the rest of the ingredients.
5. After which you stir to mix perfectly, and taste.
6. At this point, you adjust flavors to your liking.
7. Finally, you pour mixture into custard cups, ramekins, or glasses.
8. After which you chill completely (Note that it will take 3 to 4 hours until completely set).

Suggestion on how to Serve:
1. I suggest you serve with fresh or frozen berries, or without a simple berry sauce.

2. However, for the raspberry sauce, I suggest you simply thaw frozen raspberries and sweeten to taste.
3. You may strain the seeds out by forcing the berries through a strainer.
4. Other berry sauces are, sugar-free strawberry topping and easy three berry sauce.

Nutritional value: per serving
Amount per serving
Calories: 336
Carb: 3g
Protein: 3g
Fat: 35g

2.22. Raspberry Fool
Ingredients:
2 cups of heavy cream
A Sugar substitute to taste
Approximately 5 cups of raspberries (you can use frozen, thawed)
2 and 1 teaspoons of vanilla extract
Directions:
1. First, you put 2 cups of raspberries in the blender or food processor.
2. After which you add sweetener to your taste.
3. Then you whip cream with vanilla and about 2 Tablespoons of sugar equivalent.
4. For a nice presentation, I suggest you put a Tablespoon or so of raspberry puree in the bottom of a wine glass or clear dessert dish.
5. After which you mix the rest of the puree in with the whipped cream, but do not mix it too well.
6. Then you spoon into dessert dishes and garnish with the rest of the raspberries (or preferable mix some completely berries into the fool).

Nutritional value: per serving
Amount per serving
Calories: 200
Carb: 5g
Dietary fiber: 4g

2.23. Raspberry Lemon Mousse
Ingredients:
2 cups of heavy cream
2 recipe of lemon curd, chilled
3 teaspoon of vanilla extract
3 cups of fresh raspberries (you can either use frozen, but use a little less)
Sugar substitute equal to 4-6 tablespoons of sugar (liquid sucralose works fine)
Directions:
1. First, you whip cream with vanilla and sugar substitute.
2. After which you mesh raspberries with a little sweetener (or you use a blender or food processor for this purpose).
3. Then you mix cream, raspberries, and lemon curd.
4. At this point, you adjust sweetener, if you would prefer to add a bit (it all depends upon how tangy you want your mousse).
5. After which you serve in a dessert dishes, or if you want to be fancy, I suggest you use wine or martini glasses.
6. Then you garnish with raspberries.

Nutritional value: per serving
Amount per serving
Calories: 206
Carb: 3g
Protein: 4g
Dietary fiber: 1.5g

2.24. Raspberry Vanilla Cream
Tips:
1. This recipe is deluxe with a sprinkling of macadamia nuts.
2. Moreover, is good for breakfast, too!

Ingredients:
2 cups of ricotta cheese (note that whole milk type has fewest carbs and least grainy)
An Artificial sweetener equal to ½ cup of sugar, or to taste
2 cups of raspberries (frozen without sugar)
1 Tablespoon of vanilla
¼ cups of sugar free raspberry syrup (preferably Da Vinci, or raspberry flavoring plus sweetener)

Directions:
1. First, you put the raspberries and liquid in food processor or blender.
2. After which you process until mostly smooth.
3. Then you add ricotta and process until blended.
4. Finally, you refrigerate covered.

Nutritional value: per serving
Amount per serving
Calories: 146
Carb: 4g
Protein: 8g
Dietary fiber: 2g

2.25. Strawberry Daiquiri
Tips:
1. You can make this sugar-free recipe without the rum for a summer drink for adults or kids.
2. In the other hand, you can use frozen strawberries instead of the fresh and ice, but use a little less if you do not like the carb count to increase.
3. Traditionally daiquiris are prepared with lime juice, but lemon juice still tastes nice.

Ingredients:
2 Tablespoon of lime juice
1 cup of sliced strawberries
2 jigger rum (1.5 oz.)
2 Small handful of ice (it is not needed if berries are frozen)
Sweetener to taste (it depends on how sweet the strawberries are)
Directions:
First, you put in blender and push the button.
Nutritional value: per serving
Amount per serving
Calories: 125
Carb: 5g
Dietary fiber: 2g

2.26. Sweet and Sour Lime Dressing
Tips:
I prefer to whisk this right in the salad bowl, put the salad on top, and toss.
Ingredients:
2 t of water
Seasonings to taste
2 T of lime juice (from a bottle is ok)
Sweetener to taste
4 T of extra virgin olive oil
Preparation:
1. First, you put lime juice and water in bowl.
2. After which you add sweetener to the tanginess level you want.
3. Then you add salt and pepper. On the other hand, use a blend, like homemade seasoning salt.
4. At this point you whisk together to dissolve the salt.
5. After which you whisk in the olive oil.

2.27. Spinach Dip
Tips:
In this recipe, you do not have to use a food processor, but it does break the spinach down more for a smoother dip.
NOTE:
If you wish to reduce the carbs, I suggest you replace up to half of the sour cream with regular mayonnaise.
Ingredients:
3 cups of sour cream
2 10 oz. package frozen chopped spinach (thawed and squeezed dry)
Seasoning:
Either you use 8 teaspoons of a salad seasoning such as Penzey's Buttermilk Ranch
OR
1-teaspoon of garlic powder
½ teaspoon of black pepper
4 teaspoons of onion powder
1 teaspoon of salt
1 teaspoon of some kind of powdered herb, such as the Greek seasoning
Directions:
1. If you are using a food processor, I suggest you pulse the spinach alone a few times.
2. After which you add the rest of the ingredients and blend well.
3. However, if you are not using a food processor, I will also suggest you stir to combine the ingredients in a bowl.
4. Finally, when serving I suggest you serve with a vegetable dip, or spread for cucumber rounds or other vegetables.

Nutritional value:
Amount per serving
Carb: 22g
Protein: 20g
Dietary fiber: 9g

2.28. Coconut Raspberry Muffins
Tips:
First, you heat oven to a temperature of 375° F.
Make sure you prepare pan with a generous amount of butter.
This recipe is made-up of coconut flour, which has a mild coconut taste.
You can also use blueberries or raspberries.
Ingredients:
2/3 cup of coconut flour
1 teaspoon of vanilla
½ cup of sugar substitute equivalent (I prefer liquid)
1 cup of raspberries or blueberries (whichever one)
6 eggs (room temperature – very essential)
½ cup of melted butter
½ teaspoon of salt
1 teaspoon of baking powder
4-10 Tablespoons of water
Directions:
1. First, you whisk or beat the eggs until whites and yolks are well mixed.
2. After which you stream in the butter while continuing to whisk.
3. Then you add salt and vanilla and mix until combined. (NOTE: If you using liquid sweetener, I suggest you add it at this point).
4. Furthermore, you mix the remaining dry ingredients (such as the coconut flour, baking soda, and sweetener if using powder).
5. After which you mix the dry and wet ingredients together.
6. Then you now whisk in the water, one tablespoon at a time.
7. Note that the coconut flour will absorb the liquid from the wet ingredients.
8. Nevertheless, if you want to get it to a consistency that will hold up the berries, but not be too thick. I suggest you end up using about 9 Tablespoons of water.
9. Finally, you gently mix in the berries and divide among 12 muffin cups.
10. Then you bake for approximately 15 to 18 minutes or until it turns golden on top.

Nutritional value:
Amount per serving
Calories: 132
Carb: 2g
Protein: 4g
Dietary fiber: 3.5g

2.29. Cashew cheese recipe
Ingredients:
2 cups of raw or roasted cashews (260g)
4 turns fresh black pepper
½ cup water (60ml)
4 teaspoons lemon juice (10ml)
½-teaspoon salt
Tips:
1. While processing remember to turn off the food processor as you scrape down the mixture from the side (turn off the processor before you carry this out).
2. Meanwhile, soak the cashew for at least 1 hour or better still 24 hours (because the longer you soak, the creamier it will become).

Directions:
1. After you must have soaked, drained and rinsed the two cups of cashews.

2. Pour the entire ingredient into a food processor; give it a minute for the ingredients to incorporate.

3. Then you add water; allow it to stay for 2-4 minute, until it is completely smooth.

Nutritional value:
Amount per serving: 1 serving size
Calories: 168
Fat: 12.9g
Carbohydrate: 10.7g
Dietary fiber: 1.3g
Protein: 4.6g

2.30. SPINACH WITH PINE NUTS RECIPE
Ingredients:
2 teaspoons minced garlic
A freshly ground black pepper
6 pounds spinach
4 teaspoons olive oil
4 tablespoons toasted pine nut
Tips:
1. Wash the spinach thoroughly leaving a cling of water on the leaves.
2. Preheat the oil on a medium-high heat level.

Directions:
1. First, pour the spinach over boiling water, tightly covered and cook for 3 minutes over a medium-high heat, until it wilt.
2. Add the spinach, pine nuts, and garlic and cook for 2 minutes.
3. Season with pepper and serve.

Nutritional value:
Amount per serving: serving size 1 cup
Calories: 127
Fat: 10g
Carbs: 3g
Dietary fiber: 4g
Sugar: 0g
Protein: 6g
Salt: 0.84g

2.31. HAZELNUT COOKIES RECIPES

Ingredient:
4 eggs (beaten)
4 cups of toasted hazelnut
2 cups packed brown sugar
2-teaspoon vanilla extract

Tips:
1. Preheat the oven to a temperature level of 350*F.
2. Line a baking sheet with parchment paper.

Note:
1. This recipe is a clear indication that cookies do not need any flour before it called a cookie.
2. Brown sugar and groundnuts make for a wonderful cookie that any kid or adult will cherish.

DIRECTIONS:
1. First, grind the hazelnut in a food processor until coarse.
2. Then you transfer into a large bowl, add eggs, vanilla and sugar then you beat well.
3. Drop batter by the tablespoon onto prepared baking sheet; give an inch space between each cookie.
4. Finally, you bake for approximately 20 to 23 minutes, until the cookies are dark golden and firm.
5. Then you can now remove the cookies from the oven and allow cooling before removing from baking sheet.

Nutritional value:
Amount per serving
Calories: 88
Fat: 5g
Cholesterol: 0mg
Carbohydrate: 10g
Dietary fiber: 1g

Protein: 2g
Sodium: 46mg

2.32. Turkey or Chicken Tetrazzini
NOTE:
1. You can make this recipe with either spaghetti squash or shirataki noodles, or any low-carb noodle of your choice.
2. However, you can still use leftover chicken or turkey.

Ingredients:
½ cup of chopped onion
4 Tablespoons of oil or butter (or you may use ½ of each)
1 cup of cream
Salt (begin with a teaspoon, or 2 Tablespoons chicken or turkey soup base such as Better than Bouillon)
2/3 cup of dry sherry
½ cup of almond meal or low-carb bread crumbs
6 cups of cooked chopped chicken or turkey meat
16 oz. of sliced mushrooms
3 cups of unsweetened soy milk (or see note below)
Flour or other thickener of your choice
Pepper to taste
½ cup of grated Parmesan cheese

Tips prior to the preparations:
1. First, you need 4 cups of white sauce for this dish.
2. The thickener and dairy in this dish are up to you to (I use 3 cups unsweetened soy milk or unsweetened almond milk and 1 cup cream).
3. Better still you can use all milk or whatever is best for your own eating plan.
4. As for the thickener, I suggest you use 4 Tablespoons of flour and 2 Tablespoon commercial low carb thickener.

Directions for the spaghetti squash:
1. First, you prepare a spaghetti squash and take out enough strands to fill the bottom of a 9 X 13 pan.
2. I figured on 11 cups tightly packed (but I did not measure).

Directions for the Shirataki Noodles:
1. First, you use 6 packages of the spaghetti type shirataki noodles.
2. After which you rinse well in a colander, and cut into pieces with scissors.
3. Then you drain very well (I suggest you spread them on a paper towel to dry, though this might be overkill because they contain a lot of moisture).
4. Finally, you put in 9 X 13 pan or other casserole dish.

Directions for Other Types of Noodles:
1. **First, you** prepare according to package directions and add carb count to the basic recipe.
2. After which you put in 9X13 pan or other casserole dish.
3. Make sure you heat oven to a temperature of 450 F.

General directions:
1. First, you have to sauté the onions in the oil or butter.
2. After which you add the mushrooms and cook until they have given up most of their moisture.
3. Then you add salt and pepper and stir thoroughly.
4. If you are using flour for thickener, I suggest you add it here, and cook for 1 to 2 minutes.
5. After which you add liquid and other thickeners, and bring to a simmer.
6. Then you add the sherry, if you wish to.
7. Furthermore, you add the turkey, and bring back to a simmer.
8. At this point you mix with noodles or squash in casserole pan.
9. Finally, you sprinkle almond meal and cheese on top.
10. Then you bake for approximately 10 minutes, or until topping begins to brown.

Nutritional value:
Amount per serving
Calories: 232

Carb: 3.5g
Protein: 21g
Dietary fiber: 1g

2.33. Cauliflower Cheese Soup

Tips:
1. This soup is awesome with ham in it, or greens.
2. To make without cornstarch is not that bad, it is just less good, especially on reheating.
3. I recommend you use about half the amount of cheese (or no cheese) because the soup is actually quite good as a creamy cauliflower soup.
4. You might feel like adding a touch more cream in that case.

Ingredients:
1 medium onion (chopped about 4 oz.)
4 cups of chicken stock or broth (or 4 cups water with chicken base such as Better than Bouillon)
1 teaspoon of dried thyme (or 1 tablespoon of fresh thyme)
½ teaspoon of paprika (you may add a nice rosy color)
½ cup of heavy cream
1-tablespoon of cornstarch
1 large head of cauliflower (approximately 7 inches in diameter, broken or chopped up into roughly equal florets)
5 cloves of garlic (pressed, grated, or minced fine)
Add 3 bay leaves
Pinch cayenne (or other hot pepper)
½ lb. of cheddar cheese (preferable white)
1 tablespoon of mustard (either yellow or brown)
Add salt and pepper to taste

Directions:
1. First, you heat the oil and cook the onion in a large pot or Dutch oven (best if it holds about 3 quarts), until it begins to soften, approximately 4 or 5 minutes.
2. After which you add garlic, and cook another 30 seconds or thereabout.
3. Then you add the cauliflower, and stir.

4. Furthermore, you add the chicken broth; herbs and spices then you cover, and bring to a simmer.
5. After which you cook until the cauliflower is soft, approximately 10 minutes.
6. Then you remove bay leaves.
7. At this point while the vegetables are cooking, you grate the cheese, and toss with the cornstarch.
8. Then when the cauliflower is soft, you puree the soup with an immersion (stick) blender if you have one.
9. If you do not have one, I suggest you puree in batches in a regular stand blender, but be careful not to blend too much at a time (note that hot liquids can "explode" when blended and spewing hot liquid all over the place).
10. Finally, you add the cream and the cheese and stir as the cheese melts.
11. After which you add the mustard (
12. At this point, make sure you taste and adjust salt and spices.
13. Then you garnish with chives or bacon crumbles.

Nutritional value:
Amount per serving
Calories: 215
Carb: 7g
Protein: 10g
Dietary fiber: 3g

2.34. Fajitas - Chicken or Beef
Tips:
Feel free to use whatever beef of your choice, or boneless skinless chicken breast.
Ingredients:
2 medium onion, sliced, or 30 medium scallions (preferable green onions) - same amount of carb!
½ cup of soy sauce
3 ½ lbs. of skirt steak (or other beef or chicken easily cut into strips)
4 large Bell peppers (sliced preferably 2 different colors would be nice)
½ cup of lime juice
4 Tablespoons of oil
2 teaspoons of chili powder
Directions:
1. First, you combine the soy sauce, lime juice, chili powder, and oil.
2. If you are grilling, I suggest you save a couple of Tablespoons aside to toss with the vegetables.
3. After which you slice the meat into about ½-inch slices.
4. If you using skirt steak, flank steak, or other meat with an obvious grain (I mean lines through the meat), I suggest you make sure you cut perpendicular to the grain.
5. However, if you cooking in a skillet, I suggest you marinate everything together in a bowl or plastic bag (preferable a zip-type).
6. In the other hand, if you are grilling, I suggest you marinate the meat and veggies separately.
7. If grilling, I suggest you remove from marinade and grill.
8. As for cooking in a skillet (prefer the regular and not the nonstick), cook the meat first (it will probably take two batches, it all depends upon your pan).
9. Finally, you add a little oil to the skillet and get it very hot (the oil will shimmer).
10. Note that the meat will steam instead of browning, if you do not get it hot enough (or crowd too much meat in).
11. When the meat is brown and begin to soften, I suggest you remove and add veggies then you return to the skillet to heat through.
12. Then you can now serve with salsa, sour cream, and cilantro (if you so wished) and guacamole (Note: If you have low-carb tortillas, feel free to use, because it will make a nice addition, but a fork works fine).

Nutritional value:
Amount per serving
Calories: 307
Carb: 4.5g
Protein: 28g
Dietary fiber: 2g

2.35. Fresh Berry Pie
Tips:
1. I suggest you make this pie with fresh blackberries or raspberries. (My very favorite for this recipe is the olallieberry, a variety of blackberry that grows near the West Coast of the United States.)
2. Note that the filling is mostly uncooked, with just a glaze for the fresh berries. I suggest you use the almond pie crust for this recipe.

Ingredients:
2 quart (8 cups) fresh blackberries
1 ½ cup of water
2 Tablespoon of butter (it is optional, but recommended)
You could use 1 ½ cups of Da Vinci's Simple Syrup instead of water
2 almond pie crust, baked (see link above)
2 Dash of salt
Sugar substitute to taste (approximately 1 ½ cups of liquid form of Splenda preferred)
8 teaspoons of corn starch

Directions:
1. First, you mix the water, two cups of berries, salt, and sweetener in a saucepan (Note: it should be big enough to eventually hold all the berries).
2. After which you bring the mixture to a boil and cook for approximately 2 to 3 minutes.
3. Make sure berries are softening and the liquid berry-colored.
4. Then you whisk cornstarch into mixture.
5. You have to make sure it is well dissolving, then you cook until mixture darkens and clarifies (most of the lightness from the cornstarch will go away).
6. Furthermore, you add butter, and stir until melted.
7. After which you add the rest of the berries, and stir until coated with the glaze.
8. Finally, you pour into baked shell and chill.
9. Then you top with whipped cream flavored with a bit of vanilla and sweetener, before you serve.

Nutritional value: per serving
Amount per serving
Calories: 189
Carb: 5.5g
Protein: 6g
Dietary fiber: 6g

2.36. Lasagna in a Bowl
Tips:
1. This recipe can be made into spinach lasagna, eggplant lasagna, zucchini lasagna, etc. This you can achieve by putting a vegetable layer in over the meat.
2. You can use any kind of whole-grain pasta, which is if your diet allows.

NOTE: This recipe is easily adaptable to family members with varieties of tastes and nutritional needs.
Ingredients:
For Per Serving:
½ Cup of spaghetti sauce (sugar-free)
A ground meat, cooked and drained (1 lb. makes approximately 6 servings)
1/3 Cup of ricotta cheese
¼ Cup of shredded mozzarella cheese
1 Cup of cooked spaghetti squash (or other low carb pasta alternative)
2 Tablespoons of parmesan cheese
Directions:
1. First you cook the "pasta substitute", be it spaghetti squash or something else.
2. After which you cook the meat with salt and pepper to taste.
3. Then you drain off the fat.
4. You can combine the sauce and the meat at this point, i.e. if you wish.
5. Then you heat the ricotta (microwave works well) For the Layer in bowl: this are the pasta alternative, ricotta cheese, ground meat, mozzarella, sauce, parmesan.

Nutritional value (with spaghetti squash): per serving
Amount per serving
Carb: 19g
Protein: 38g

Dietary fiber: 3g

2.37. Lemon Mousse
Tips:
1. This recipe is a combination of whipped cream with sugar-free lemon curd.
2. I advise you not to try it with a commercial sugar-free lemon curd, because you might be disappointed.

Ingredients:
2 recipe lemon curd, chilled (see instruction above)
1 ¼ cup of heavy cream, preferably not ultra-pasteurized
2 teaspoons of vanilla extract
A sugar substitute equal to 2-3 tablespoons sugar (liquid sucralose works best)
Directions:
1. First, you whip cream with vanilla and sugar substitute.
2. After which you mix with lemon curd.
3. Then you adjust sweetener if you would like to add a little (it all depends upon how tangy you want your mousse).
4. Finally, you serve in dessert dishes, or if you want to be fancy, wine or martini glasses.

Garnish with berries or mint.
Nutritional value: per serving
Amount per serving
Calories: 209
Carb: 2g
Protein: 4g

2.38. No-Bake Cheesecake
Tips:
1. You can top this recipe in many different ways.
2. The crust requires a few minutes in the oven, but you can also serve it crust less.
3. The easiest topping for this recipe is to spread a jar of sugar-free jam over it.
4. It would add approximately 2 grams of carb per serving to the basic cheesecake.
5. Other alternative are to top with fresh fruit in season, I suggest strawberry topping, or simply cook frozen berries with sweetener to taste until thickened.

Ingredients:
10 oz. of cream cheese (room temperature)
1 teaspoon of lemon juice
1 cup of heavy cream
1 almond pie crust
2 teaspoons of vanilla extract
Zero-carb sugar substitute (preferable, liquid sucralose) equal to approximately ½ cup of sugar (or to taste)

Directions:
1. First, you bake the almond piecrust, in either a deep-dish pie pan or spring form pan.
2. NOTE: if you using a pie pan, you do not need to spread the crust to the rim of the pan.
3. After which you mix thoroughly cream cheese, vanilla, lemon juice, and sugar substitute.
4. If you are using an electric mixer, I suggest you fluff it up for a minute or two.
5. In a second bowl, but if you have only one bowl for a stand mixer, I suggest just transfer the cream cheese and use the mixer again for this step.
6. At this point, you whip the cream to soft peaks (you might actually want it slightly less beaten than you would for a dessert topping).
7. Then you mix about a third of the whipped cream into the cream cheese mixture.
8. After which you gently mix another third in, and then the rest.
9. Finally, you spread cream cheese mixture into crust.

10. After which you Smooth off and chill for approximately 2-3 hours.
11. Then you cover with topping and serve.

Crestless alternative:
1. First, you chill cream cheese mixture in bowl.
2. After which you serve in individual dishes with topping.

Lower-calorie alternative:
1. Initially, use low fat or fat-free cream cheese (I suggest you add an extra gram or two of carb)
2. After which you mix the crust.

Nutritional value: per serving
Amount per serving
Calories: 230
Carb: 2g
Protein: 7g

2.39. Peanut Butter Protein Balls
Tips:
1. Remember, that in the recipe the exact ratio of ingredients all depends a little on the kinds of protein powder and peanut butter you use taste.
2. I suggest a designer Protein, French Vanilla flavor, for this basic recipe, but chocolate and other flavors also works well.
3. If the peanut butter has more oil (natural peanut butters will vary quite a bit for oil content), I suggest you will probably need more protein powder.
4. In addition, the quantity of sweetener is obviously to taste.
5. Have it in mind that these balls are soft at room temperature, so therefore you cannot throw them in a bag and expect that they will hold their shape.

Ingredients:
8 scoops (or 2 and 2/3 cups) whey protein powder (most are low in carbs, but check any flavor)
Artificial sweetener to taste (approximately 2-3 cups of sugar equivalent)
2 cups of peanut butter (sugar-free)
2 teaspoons of vanilla extract
Directions:
1. First, you put the entire ingredients in a mixing bowl and mix all at once.
2. I recommend you use mixer because it works great for this, but a food processor would probably be fine as well, or just a spoon.
3. After which you roll into balls.
4. Roll in crushed nuts, If you so wish.
5. I suggest you use mixed almond meal with powdered erythritol as your coating.
6. For your sweetener, I suggest you use the most concentrated liquid sucralose (Splenda).

Nutritional value: per serving
Amount per serving
Calories: 118
Carb: 3g
Protein: 9g

Dietary fiber: 1g

2.40. Pimento Cheese Spread
Tips:
You can substitute roasted red pepper for the pimento.
Ingredients for 4 oz. cream cheese, at room temperature
2 (4 oz.) jar pimentos, or 1 roasted red pepper
2 hot sauce to taste (it is optional)
2 (8 oz.) cheddar cheese (I prefer to use a combination of white and yellow cheddar)
8 Tablespoons of mayonnaise
2 Tablespoons of prepared mustard
Directions:
1. First, you cut cheese into chunks of approximately 1 inch, and pulse in food processor (or you can use grated cheese).
2. After which you add the rest of the ingredients and blend until smooth.
3. Then you taste and adjust if it is a little harsh.

If possible, I suggest you try rounding it out with a very small amount of sweetener (like a drop of a concentrated liquid sucralose sweetener).
Nutritional value: per serving
Amount per serving
Calories: 98
Carb: 1/2 g
Protein: 1g

2.41. Pumpkin Cheesecake
Tips
1. Meanwhile, you heat oven to 375 F.
2. After which you prepare spring form pan: I prefer to place a piece of parchment paper over the bottom of the pan.
3. There is no need to cut it to size, just snap it into place when you put the tighten the sides.
4. Then you wrap the bottom and sides of the pan in heavy-duty foil.
5. You are going to be baking the cheesecake with the spring form pan set in a baking pan half-full of boiling water, so to protect from leaks.

Note:
1. This version of pumpkin cheesecake is richly spiced.
2. The crust is thicker than the regular low-carb cheesecake, but if you want a thinner crust, I will advise you use the other one.
3. If you prefer a cheesecake that is not as rich, I suggest you use lower fat cream cheese (though I have not specifically tried it with more than one package of the cream cheese being low-fat).

Ingredients:
Ingredient for the crust:
1 teaspoon of each of ginger and cinnamon
8 Tablespoons of sugar substitute
3 cups of almond meal
8 Tablespoons of melted butter
Ingredient for the Filling:
6 (8 oz.) of packages cream cheese at room temperature
5 teaspoons of cinnamon
2 teaspoons of nutmeg
1 ½ teaspoons of ginger
½ teaspoon of allspice
½ teaspoon of cloves

1 teaspoon of salt
3 cups of sugar substitute (or to taste, preferable liquid sucralose as it is zero carb)
2 cans (about 15 oz.) of pumpkin
2 Tablespoons of vanilla
10 eggs (preferably room temperature)
1 cup of heavy cream

Directions:
1. First, you combine the ingredients for crust, and press into the bottom of a spring form pan.
2. After which you bake for about 8 to 10 minutes, until fragrant and beginning to brown.
3. Then you beat cream cheese until fluffy.
4. Furthermore, you scrape sides of bowl and beaters.
5. Make sure you repeat this step several times, because it essential.
6. You will observe that the mixture will gradually become lighter, and the denser stuff has a tendency to cling to the bowl.
7. Keep scraping, because you might not be able to incorporate it as well later.
8. At this point, you add spices and sweetener.
9. After which you beat again, scrape again.
10. Then you add pumpkin and vanilla. Beat well, and scrape.
11. Also, add 3 eggs. Beat well (about a minute later), and scrape.
12. In addition, you add the other 2 eggs and cream and beat another minute.
13. After that, you pour mixture into pan over crust.
14. Then you place pan in a baking pan and pour boiling water around the sides, approximately halfway up.
15. You then lower the oven temperature to 325 F and bake for about 60 to 90 minutes, checking often after an hour.
16. At this point, when the cake is firm to touch but slightly soft in the center, or the center reaches 150 to 155 F, I suggest you remove from oven.
17. Finally, you remove sides from pan.
18. After which you let the cheesecake cool to room temperature, or up to 3 hours.
19. Then you cover and chill, ideally for another 3 to 4 hours.

Nutritional value: per serving
Amount per serving
Calories: 285

Carb: 4g
Protein: 5g
Dietary fiber: 2g

2.42. Sweet and Sour Mix
Tips:
1. In this recipe, you can vary the concentrations of the juices and sweetener, according to your taste, the particular juices you use, and how much you want your ice to be.
2. Note that you can use this mix to make daiquiris; whiskey sours, margaritas, etc. (I suggest you eat it with Jack Daniels).
3. Limes and Fresh lemon taste good, but bottled one works fine.

Ingredients:
½ cup of lemon juice
½ cup of equivalent artificial sweetener (preferable liquid)
2 cups of water
4 Tablespoons of lime juice
Directions:
1. First, you combine the entire ingredient together.
2. After which you store covered in the refrigerator.

Nutritional value: per cup of mixer
Amount per serving
Carb: 6g
3. Taco Salad

Tips:
1. This version of recipe is easy to throw together when you do not feel like cooking, especially if you have the meat prepared ahead of time.
2. I suggest you "dress" the salad individually with the sour cream and salsa.
3. However, if you like more dressing, I suggest a low-carb ranch type or a lemon and olive oil dressing.

Ingredients:
8 green onions (chopped and it's white and green parts separated into two piles)
A Salt and pepper to taste
1 medium tomato, chopped
A small can (4 oz.) chopped or sliced ripe olives (it is optional)
1 pound of ground beef
1 tablespoon of chili powder
1 head of romaine lettuce (chopped)
1 avocado (diced)
1 ½ cups of grated cheese (cheddar, Monterey Jack, or a combination of both)
½ cup of salsa
½ cup of sour cream
Directions:
1. First, you cook the beef in skillet with chili powder, white part of onions, and salt and pepper.
2. After which you put in the salad warm or chilled, as you prefer.
3. Then you mix the lettuce, tomato, avocado, green onion, and olives.
4. Finally, you add the meat and cheese and toss together.
5. After which you put it on top of each individual serving.
6. Then you top with salsa and sour cream.

Nutritional value: each of 5 serving
Amount per serving
Calories: 505
Carb: 5.5g
Protein: 36g
Dietary fiber: 4g

3.1. Crock Pot Chicken Cacciatore
Tips:
1. This dish is a bit tricky in the crock-pot, this is because the water tends to come out of the vegetables and make the sauce too thin.
2. This is the sole reason why I sauté the vegetables beforehand, reduce the liquid, and add tomato paste. It will speed the cooking time.

Ingredients:
1 cup of onion (chopped)
8 oz. of brown crimini or Portobello mushrooms (roughly chopped)
1 teaspoon of olive oil
2/3 cup of dry wine (either you use white or red)
Salt and pepper to taste
1 inch of Parmesan cheese rind (it is optional)
3 lbs. of skinless chicken thighs and/or legs (bone-in; but if you are using boneless, 8 or 9 thighs)
1 green bell pepper, medium size (chopped)
4 cloves of garlic
1 can of tomatoes, chopped (it should be about 14 oz.)
1 Tablespoon of Italian seasoning mixture (or 1 teaspoon each of oregano, basil, and thyme)
1/3 cup of tomato paste
Directions:
1. First, you season the chicken with the salt and pepper.
2. After which you put in crock-pot set to high, and cover.
3. In the other hand, you can brown the chicken before or after you removing the skin.
4. Then you pour off most of the fat before cooking the vegetables.

5. Furthermore, you cook the onion and green pepper in a large skillet with a small quantity of oil on high heat.
6. After about 2 to 3 minutes, then you add the mushrooms.
7. Then two minutes later, you then add the garlic.
8. After which you cook for another minute.
9. At this point, you add the tomatoes, wine, herbs, and more salt and pepper.
10. After which you boil for 5 to 10 minutes, until liquid completely boiled away.
11. Then you taste and adjust seasonings, if necessary.
12. Remember If it tastes harsh or acidic, I suggest you add just a touch of sweetener (preferably, one drop of Sweet free can do the trick).
13. Finally, you add the tomato paste and Parmesan cheese rind, and stir to combine.
14. After which you spoon ingredients onto the top of the chicken, and cook for about 3 hours on high or 6 to 8 hours on low.
15. Then when it is about half an hour before you are ready to eat, I suggest you check and adjust seasonings one more time.

Nutritional value: each of 6 serving
Amount per serving
Calories: 178
Carb: 10g
Protein: 20g
Dietary fiber: 3g

3.2. Denver Casserole
Note:
1. This recipe is great as a main dish for dinner or brunch.
2. Remember that the leftovers make a nice quick breakfast.
3. I prefer to put whatever vegetables I need to use up in this casserole.
4. I recommend this recipe for South Beach dieters.
5. However, for those desiring a lower-calorie option, I suggest you use low or nonfat versions of the ingredients (obviously, the calorie count will be low).

Tips:
Meanwhile, you heat oven to a temperature of 350 F.

Ingredients:
1-pint (16 oz.) of sour cream
1 lb. of cooked ham, chopped (check to be sure it is not loaded with sugar)
¼ Cup of chopped onion
Salt and pepper to taste
1 dozen of eggs
12 oz. of shredded cheese (preferable jack and/or cheddar)
1 large green pepper (chopped)
2 cloves of garlic (it is optional)

Directions:
1. First, you Sauté the onion, pepper, and garlic until it begins to soften.
2. After which you put the eggs and sour cream in blender with salt and pepper, or whisk in a bowl.
3. Then you blend very well.
4. Furthermore, you put half the cheese into a 9X13 baking pan or a similarly size casserole dish.
5. After which you add the ham next, then the rest of the cheese, and the vegetables.
6. At this point, you pour the egg mixture over the whole thing.

Finally, you bake for about 50-60 minutes, until top is golden brown and knife inserted into the center comes out clean (Note that it will continue to cook for a few minutes afterwards). **Nutritional value: per 8 servings**
Amount per serving
Calories: 533
Carb: 4.5g
Protein: 30g
Dietary fiber: 0.5g

3.3. Easy Blue Cheese Dressing
Tips:
1. Remember that you can whip this blue cheese dressing up in two minutes.
2. You have no reason to pour the watered-down bottled dressing with very little blue cheese in it on your lovely salad!
3. Do not worry if you do not have garlic powder or Worcestershire sauce, but they really do make a difference in the dressing.

Ingredients:
1 cup of sour cream
1 Tablespoon of apple cider (or wine vinegar)
1/2 teaspoon of garlic powder (it is optional)
1 cup of regular mayonnaise
6 oz. of blue cheese
2 teaspoons of Worcestershire sauce (it is optional)
½ teaspoon of pepper
Directions:
1. First, you crumble the blue cheese.
2. After which you mix it all together.
3. Then you thin with water if you so wished.

Nutritional value: per serving
Amount per serving
Calories: 135
Carb: ½ g
Protein: 2g

3.4. Super-Easy Guacamole
Ingredients:
Approximately ¼ teaspoon of salt per avocado
Approximately 3/4 t garlic powder per avocado
Chopped cilantro, chopped onion (it is Optional)
Avocados (the number should be according to the size of the crowd)
Approximately 2 Tablespoons of salsa per avocado
Approximately ½ teaspoons of lemon or lime juice per avocado
Directions:
1. First, you cut the avocados in half, squeeze out the pit (squeeze gently until it pops out).
2. After which you scoop the fruit into a bowl.
3. Then you add the salt, juice, salsa, and garlic powder.
4. Furthermore, you mash it together with a fork (I prefer leaving some chunks).
5. At this point, you taste, but if you cannot taste the avocado much, I suggest you add a bit of salt.
6. In the other hand, if it is a little flat, I suggest you dribble a little juice in.
7. If it is not spicy enough, I suggest you add a little salsa.
8. After which you try more garlic powder to see how that changes it.
9. Then you play with it and you will find an "ideal guacamole balance point" (secret to excellent guacamole!)
10. In addition, you stir in cilantro and onion at the end if you wish to.
11. By the third time, you do this, I assure you that you will not bother to measure; you will just put the ingredients in and start tasting.
12. For a healthy low-carb snack, I suggest you serves with vegetables such as cucumber, pepper strips, jicama.

Nutritional value: per serving
Amount per serving
Carb: 3g
Dietary fiber: 12g

3.5. EASY Chocolate Peanut Butter Fudge
Tips:
1. This recipe is much better if you use powdered erythritol as part of the sweetener.
2. I also think Xylitol might work well too.
3. Descriptions on how to do the sweeteners is stated bellow.
4. This fudge is intense so I suggest you cut it into even smaller squares, as a little really satisfies.

Ingredients:
1 cup of smooth peanut butter (with no added sugar)
1 cup of sugar-equivalent (of other zero-carb sugar substitute such as liquid sucralose)
A Pinch salt
8 oz. of unsweetened chocolate squares (see note)
¾ to 1 cup of erythritol
½ teaspoon of vanilla
Directions:
1) Melt the chocolate. I like to pour boiling water over it, let it sit for 5 to 6 minutes, and then pour the water off. That way I know I will not burn the chocolate. 2) Mix in the rest of the ingredients, adjusting sweetener to taste. 3) Pack or spread into a loaf pan. Cool to room temperature, or you can put it in the refrigerator. Cut into 18 pieces and serve.
Nutritional value: per serving
Amount per serving
Calories: 146
Carb: 3g

Protein: 5g
Dietary fiber: 3g

3.6. Easy Shrimp Scampi
Ingredients:
2-3 cloves of garlic (crushed)
2 Tablespoons of dry white wine (or vermouth)
1 Tablespoon of butter
2 Tablespoons of minced shallots (it is optional)
1 lb. of raw shelled deveined shrimp
2 Tablespoons of lemon juice (I prefer it fresh)
1 Tablespoon of olive oil
A Salt and Pepper
1-2 Tablespoons of minced parsley (it is optional)
The Zest of one lemon (it is optional)
A pinch of cayenne pepper (or red pepper flakes, note that it is optional)
Directions:
1. First, you heat the skillet until it is hot.
2. However, while it is heating, salt and pepper the shrimp.
3. After which you add the oil and swirl to coat.
4. Then you add the shrimp and cook for about 1-2 minutes.
5. At this point, you stirring or turning it until it just turns pink.
6. Make sure you cook a little longer at the end, so do not worry if you are not sure whether it is ok in the middle.
7. After which you turn the heat down, and add the butter to the pan. (At this point, If you using the shallot, I suggest you cook for about a minute.)
8. Then you add the garlic and red pepper.
9. Cook until fragrant, and then add wine and lemon juice (and lemon zest if available).

10. Finally, you add the shrimp back to the pan, stir, and heat through.
11. Then you add parsley if you have it.
Nutritional value: per 6 servings
Amount per serving
Calories: 250
Carb: 3g
Protein: 31g

3.7. Egg Free Chocolate Mousse
Notes
1. Varieties of chocolate have different densities.
2. If you are using a super-dense chocolate such as Scharffenberger, I suggest you add an extra 2 tablespoons of water.
3. I suggest you use Ghirardelli unsweetened chocolate when developing the recipe.
4. I suggest you substitute sugar-free syrups such as Da Vinci with (I prefer the hazelnut), or other flavorings, adding water to make 1 tablespoon.
5. If you do not have espresso powder, I suggest you use either instant coffee, or substitute with 2 tablespoons of brewed espresso or 3 tablespoons coffee for the same amount of water in the recipe.
6. If you want a lighter mousse, I suggest you use only 2 or 3 ounces of chocolate.

Ingredients:
2 Tablespoons of unsweetened cocoa powder
½ cup of sugar substitute (or more to taste, preferably liquid)
1 teaspoon of espresso powder (see below for more detail)
One teaspoon of vanilla
1 Tablespoon of rum, brandy, or uses flavoring (see below for more detail)
1 cup of powdered erythritol (or you may use xylitol)
4 oz. of unsweetened chocolate (broken up)
1 ½ cup of heavy cream
1 pinch of salt
Directions:
1. First, you cover the chocolate with boiling water, in a large bowl.
2. **After which you** pour the water off the chocolate (you do not have to get every bit), try saving ¼ cup aside.

3. Then you stir the gelatin powder into the warm water, until it dissolves.
4. Furthermore, you add rum or flavoring and liquid sweetener, if used, to water.
5. After which you whisk cocoa, salt, and espresso powder into the chocolate, followed by the liquids.
6. Then you whip cream in a separate bowl, with a couple of drops of sweetener (or preferably a small amount of powdered), and the vanilla, until soft peaks form.
7. At this point, you mix about a 3rd of the whipped cream into the chocolate mixture to lighten it.
8. Then you fold the rest in, ½ at a time.
9. **Finally, you** spoon into individual glasses, cups, or bowls, cover, and chill for about an hour before you serving.

Nutritional value: per serving
Amount per serving
Calories: 232
Carb: 3g
Protein: 3g
Dietary fiber: 3g

3.8. Five-Minute Sweet Spiced Pecans
Tips:
This pecan can also serve greatly in salads.
Ingredients:
4 tablespoons of butter
Artificial sweetener (equal to about 6 Tablespoons of sugar)
1 teaspoon of salt
4 cups of pecan halves
8 teaspoons of cinnamon
¼ teaspoons of cayenne (or other hot pepper)
Directions:
1. First, you use a large enough skillet so that the pecans will be in one layer (A nonstick skillet works fine).
2. After which you melt the butter in the skillet.
3. Then you add the hot pepper.
4. Furthermore, if you are using liquid artificial sweetener, this is the point when you add it.
5. After which you add pecans to skillet and cook over medium heat.
6. Then you stir every 30 seconds.
7. After 2 or 3 minutes, you then stir them constantly until they **just begin** to brown.
8. Note: Pecans burn quickly, so I suggest you keep your eyes on them.
9. If the butter begins to smoke before this point, I advise you turn off the heat and call them done.
10. At this point, you stir in cinnamon, salt, and powdered sweetener, i.e. if you are using it.
11. Finally, you remove from pan and place in bowl (note that pecans can still burn sitting in the hot pan).
12. When they seem cool enough to taste, I suggest that when you adjust seasonings accordingly (that is if you want more salt or sweetener).

Nutritional value: ¼ cup of pecan
Amount per serving
Carb: 1g
Dietary fiber: 3g

3.9. Greek Lemon Garlic Salad Dressing

Tips:
1. This recipe is often made with red wine vinegar and with lemon-based, especially with garlic.
2. However, the garlic tends to mellow with time.
3. If I am using the dressing right away, I always use two cloves of garlic for a cup of dressing.
4. Nevertheless, if it is going to be around longer, I use three or four cloves.
5. This dressing is a delicious combination to almost any vegetable, drizzled over with fish or marinate chicken or meats before grilling.
6. This recipe is a great way to get more healthful olive oil into your diet.

Ingredients:
1 teaspoon of salt
4 teaspoons of Greek seasoning blend (or Greek oregano)
½ cup of lemon juice (preferably fresh)
A ground pepper to taste
2 teaspoons of Dijon or brown mustard
1 ½ cups of olive oil (preferred extra virgin)
4 garlic cloves (finely grated, pressed or finely minced)

Directions:
1. I suggest that the easiest way to do this is in a glass jar (and make sure you have your storage container as well).
2. A clean jar that held a pound of peanut butter is a perfect size, but if you do not have it, I suggest you whisk in a bowl.
3. Combine the entire ingredients except olive oil (if you are using a jar, I suggest you just shake with the lid on securely).

4. At this point, you add the olive oil.
5. If you are, using the jar put the entire thing in at once and shakes very well.
6. Nevertheless, if you using a bowl, I suggest you whisk while streaming in the olive oil.
7. Remember that the mustard will help it emulsify so it looks a little creamy and not separated.
8. Then you taste, and if it tastes too acidic (some lemons are more sour than others are), I suggest you add a little more of olive oil.
9. Feel free to adjust salt and other seasonings to your taste.

Nutritional value: per serving
Amount per serving
Calories: 94
Carb: 1/3g

3.10. Tom Special, Laura Style
Tips:
1. This version of recipe has a greater proportion of eggs, and the addition of ground coriander (and a chard over spinach).
2. The traditional versions of this recipe have 4 eggs per pound of ground beef.
3. I suggest you double everything except the eggs and refrigerate or freeze half before proceeding.
4. I suggest you have this for dinner than for breakfast.
Ingredients:
1 lb. of lean ground beef
2 cups of sliced mushrooms (I prefer using shitaki for this, but use any kind)
Two (10 oz.) package frozen or raw spinach (or one bunch spinach leaves, or chard)
4 teaspoons of Worcestershire sauce
12 eggs
4 Tablespoons of olive oil
4 cloves garlic (pressed or minced)
4 teaspoons of ground coriander (seed)
Salt and pepper (I prefer quite a lot of pepper)
A shot of hot sauce (it is optional, and not traditional)
Directions:
1. First, you get a large nonstick skillet with the oil.
2. After which you thaw the spinach, only if you are using frozen.
3. Then you cook the meat.
4. I suggest that you put in everything else except for the spinach and the eggs, when it is mostly cooked.
5. When the mushrooms are mostly cooked, I suggest you add the spinach and continue until it is all hot.

6. After which you beat eggs with a little more salt and pepper.
7. Then you add to pan and cook.
8. Sprinkle with Parmesan cheese, it is optional.
Nutritional value: per serving
Amount per serving
Calories: 392
Carb: 3g
Protein: 31g
Dietary fiber: 4.5g

3.11. Thai-Style Chicken Salad Recipe
Tips:
1. This recipe is crisp, light and refreshing, and it is sweet-and-sour dressing adds a real zing.
2. It is styled after a salad called "Banana Blossom Salad"; although the ingredients are different, but the texture and flavors are similar.
Ingredients:
3 cups of shredded Napa cabbage (you can still use regular)
1 small sweet red pepper (cut it into strips)
½ cup of chopped fresh cilantro, including the stems
1 lb. of cooked chicken breast, sliced thin (you can use any chicken meat that you like)
1/3 cup of fresh mint (chopped)
3 cups of peeled jicama (cut into strips)
Ingredient for the dressing:
2 Tablespoons of lime juice
½ cup of sugar equivalent from substitute (preferably liquid such as Sweet free)
½ teaspoon of Asian chili sauce (preferable Sriracha, or other hot sauce)
3 Tablespoons of white vinegar
2 Tablespoons of Thai fish sauce
½ teaspoons of fresh grated ginger
Ingredient for garnishing:
¼ cup of chopped peanuts
Mint leaves
Cilantro leaves

Directions:
1. First, you mix all the salad ingredients.
2. After which in a separate bowl, you mix the dressing ingredients.
3. Then you toss to combine.
4. Then you garnish as desired.

Nutritional value: each of 4 servings
Amount per serving
Calories: 297
Carb: 8g
Protein: 42g
Dietary fiber: 7g

3.12. Old-Fashioned Meat Loaf
Ingredients:
2 cups of TVP
4 cloves garlic, minced (or 1-teaspoon garlic powder)
2 teaspoons of dried thyme
1 teaspoon of black pepper
4 Tablespoons of Worcestershire sauce
2 eggs
½ cup of water or milk
4 teaspoons of salt
2 teaspoons of dried sage
2 teaspoons of dry mustard powder
½ cup of onion, finely chopped (or 1 Tablespoon of dehydrated onion flakes)
4 lbs. of ground meat (about 85% to 90% lean works well). I have used turkey, beef and combinations.
Directions:
1. First, you mix the entire ingredients together in a bowl.
2. It is very easy if you use your hand, but do not over mix.
3. After which you bake in a loaf pan, several small loaf pans, or make individual ones.
4. Make sure you bake at temperature of 350 F for approximately 1 hour for a large loaf.
5. Using a muffin-cup meatloaves cook in approximately 15 to 20 minutes.
6. To be certain that the meatloaf is ok; I suggest you insert a meat thermometer, which should reach 155 F in the center of the loaf.

7. Approximately 10 to 15 minutes before you think the meatloaf will be ok, I suggest cover it with sugar-free picante sauce.
Nutritional value: each of 8 serving
Amount per serving
Calories: 263
Carb: 2g
Protein: 30g
Dietary fiber: 2g

3.13. Toasted Pumpkin Seeds
Tips:
1. This recipe also works fine for squash seeds, including spaghetti squash.
2. If you wish to add salt or seasonings to this recipe, I suggest you will need a little oil so it will stick.
3. Meanwhile, you heat oven to a temperature of 350 F. (or see instruction below for lower slower method).
Ingredients:
Pumpkin or squash seeds
Directions:
1. First, you clean the pulp off the pumpkin seeds or squash seeds.
2. After which you let dry with paper towels.
3. Then if you so wish, toss with a little olive or other oil of your choice.
4. Remember, that you only need enough to coat it a little; otherwise, they will be greasy.
5. At this point, you add salt and any kind of seasoning you wish to use such as Cajon seasoning, garlic powder, dried Chile powder est.
6. After which you cover the baking sheet with a parchment paper.
7. Then you spread out the seeds out in a layer.
8. Finally, you bake for about 3-5 minutes, until seeds start to color and are fragrant.
9. You may use a safer method of using a lower temperature.
10. I understand that if you roast the seeds at about 250 degrees F.
11. You do not have to watch them carefully; it takes approximately 45 -60 minutes.
Nutritional value: per serving
Amount per serving

Carb: 5g
Dietary fiber: 2g

3.14. Seared Scallops

Tips:
1. This recipe is elegant, easy, quick cooking, and delicious.
2. The trick in this recipe is in quick simple preparation, so the scallops are perfectly cooked and the flavor shines through.
3. It is very easy to overcook the scallops and it can be a nice first course.

Ingredients:
2 Tablespoons of oil or butter
Salt and pepper to taste
2 pounds of sea scallops

Directions:
1. **First, you** dry the scallops with paper towels.
2. After which you salt and pepper both sides.
3. **Then you** heat a large regular pan for about 2-3 minutes so it is quite hot.
4. At this point, you add the oil or butter, and then the scallops.
5. Make sure you do not let them touch each other.
6. If your pan is not big enough to do then all at a goal, I suggest you keep the first batch under a piece of foil and do two batches.
7. After which you cook the scallops for 1½ minutes each side.
8. Make sure they have a golden crust on both ends, and the center should still look translucent.
9. Then you turn with tongs.
10. Make sure you serve immediately.

Suggestions when serving:
You can serve with greens sautéed in garlic with a squeeze of lemon, with mushrooms in garlic and wine, as part of an elegant salad (or many other ways).

Nutritional value: per serving
Amount per serving
Calories: 132
Carb: 3.5g
Protein: 25g

3.15. Strawberry Vinaigrette
Tips:
1. This dressing is nice on any green salad, I suggest you give it a trial try it for something different.
2. It is preferable with Strawberry Chicken Salad, a meal salad with greens, strawberries, and chicken.
Ingredients:
1 cup of sliced strawberries
4 tablespoons of red wine vinegar (balsamic is preferable, but carb counts vary, so be careful)
A Sweetener to taste (it solely depends on the sweetness of strawberries; you might not need it.
1 cup of olive oil
Salt and pepper to your taste
2 teaspoons of mustard
Directions:
1. First, you puree strawberries in a blender or food processor.
2. After which you add vinegar, mustard, and seasonings.
3. At this point, you blend, and then add olive oil.
4. After which you blend until creamy.
5. Then you taste and adjust seasonings.
Nutritional value: per serving
Amount per serving
Calories: 123
Carb: ½ g

3.16. Swordfish Burgers
Ingredients:
4 garlic cloves
½ cup of breadcrumbs
Salt and fresh pepper to taste
Mixed greens (or chopped romaine)
Oil spray
Lemon zest
4 shallots
3 lbs. (48 oz.) of swordfish steaks, skin removed
6 tablespoons of chopped chives
Ingredient for the Lemon Vinaigrette:
16 teaspoons of extra virgin olive oil
2 lemon (juiced)
Salt and fresh pepper to taste
Directions:
1. First, you cut fish into large chunks, and put about ¼ of the fish into a food processor along with garlic and shallots.

2. After which you pulse until it becomes almost pasty.

3. After that, you place into a medium bowl.

4. At this point, you place the remaining fish into food processor and pulse on and off until chopped.

5. Then you combine with the rest of the fish in the bowl and add chives, lemon zest, breadcrumbs, salt and pepper.

6. Furthermore, you mix well and form into 4 patties.

7. Spray a little oil in a large non-stick skillet and heat on medium-high.

8. After that, you add fish and cook for about 4 minutes on each side.

Direction to BBQ:
1. First, you grill 4-6 inches above the fire on a lightly oiled grill rack.

2. After that, you grill on medium flame, about 4 minutes on each side.

3. At this point, you whisk vinaigrette ingredients in a small bowl.

4. Then you can now serve fish burgers over a bed of greens and drizzle with lemon vinaigrette

Nutritional value:
Amount per serving: 1 serving size
Calories: 304.3
Fat: 16.0g
Carbohydrate: 5.3g
Dietary fiber: 0.7g
Protein: 33.4g

3.17. Avocado Coconut Popsicles
Ingredients:
4 ¼ cups of unsweetened Almond Breeze Almond Coconut milk
1 cup of sweetened shredded coconut flakes (preferably, Baker's)
8 oz. haas avocado (from 2 medium)
12 tablespoons of raw sugar (or preferably your favorite sweetener)
Directions:
1. First, you combine the avocado, milk and sugar in the blender and mix until smooth.

2. After which you add the coconut flakes and mix to incorporate.

3. Then you pour into the popsicle mold and freeze.

Nutritional value:
Amount per serving: 1 serving size
Calories: 84
Fat: 1g
Carbohydrate: 11g
Dietary fiber: 1g
Protein: 1g

3.18. Chocolate Ricotta Mousse
Ingredients:
6 tablespoons of unsweetened cocoa powder
Pinches of salt
4 cups of part-skim ricotta
4 large egg whites (room temperature)
1 cup of sugar
Directions:
1. First, you blend ricotta and cocoa powder until completely smooth on a food processor (or blender should work)
2. .
3. After which you transfer to a large bowl.

4. After that, you place egg whites, sugar, salt in a medium heatproof mixing bowl (metal) and place bowl on top of a pot of simmering water.

5. At this point, you cook and whisk constantly until the sugar dissolves and the mixture is warm, about 3 minutes.

6. Then you remove bowl from heat and beat with an electric mixer on high, until stiff peaks form (approximately 5 minutes).

7. This is when you gently fold egg white mixture into the bowl using a rubber spatula, with ricotta until well combined.

8. Finally, you divide into 6 6 oz. ramekins or small bowls and then refrigerate at least 3 hours.

Nutritional value:
Amount per serving: 1 serving size
Calories: 166
Fat: 7g
Carbohydrate: 18g
Dietary fiber: 1g

Protein: 11g

3.19. Raspberry Coconut Chia Pudding Pops
Ingredients:
1 cup of unsweetened almond milk
4 tablespoons of chia seeds
16 drop of Nu-Naturals liquid stevia (or preferably sugar/honey to taste)
1cup of lite coconut milk
1 ¼ cup of raspberries
2 tablespoons of sweetened shredded coconut
Directions:
1. First, you combine the entire ingredients in a large container.

2. After which you mix well and close container; then you refrigerate for 4 hours so the chia expands.

3. Then you pour into 4 Popsicle molds and freeze overnight.

Nutritional value:
Amount per serving: 1 serving size
Calories: 74
Fat: 5g
Carbohydrate: 6.8g
Dietary fiber: 4.6g
Protein: 1.8g

3.20. Avocado Egg Salad
Ingredients:
8 hardboiled egg whites (chopped, discard the rest)
2 tablespoons of light mayonnaise
1 tablespoon of finely chopped chives
Pinches of freshly ground pepper
8 large hard-boiled eggs (chopped)
2 medium hass avocado (cut into 1/2-inch pieces)
2 tablespoons of fat free plain yogurt
1 teaspoons of kosher salt
4 teaspoons of red wine vinegar
Directions:
1. First, you mix the egg yolks with the avocado, yogurt, light mayo, vinegar, salt, chives and pepper after which you mash with a fork.

2. Finally, you mix with egg whites and adjust salt to your satisfaction.

Nutritional value:
Amount per serving: 1 serving size
Calories: 154.7
Fat: 11.7g
Carbohydrate: 4.6g
Dietary fiber: 3g
Protein: 9.3g

3.21. Greek Salad Sandwich
Ingredients:
8 teaspoons of extra virgin olive oil
8 thin slices of red onion
8 tablespoons of crumbled feta
16 Romaine lettuce leaves
2 medium tomatoes (thinly sliced)
4 tablespoons of red wine vinegar
10 tablespoons of Kalamata olives (minced)
Coarse salt and fresh ground pepper
24 oz. ciabatta bread (cut into 4 pieces)
1 medium cucumber (thinly sliced)
Directions:
1. First, you whisk red wine vinegar, and olive oil, in a small bowl then you season with salt and pepper.

2. After which you add chopped olives and red onions and then you set aside.

3. I prefer adding onions to the vinegar, this mellows out the sharpness of the onion, but completely optional

4. After that, you spread the olive mixture on 4 slices bread.
5. Then you top with lettuce, cucumber, tomatoes, and red onion.

6. At this point, you season with salt and pepper.

7. Finally, you top with feta, close and cut sandwich in half

Nutritional value:
Amount per serving: 1 serving size
Calories: 291

Fat: 8g
Carbohydrate: 46g
Dietary fiber: 1.5g
Protein: 8.4g

3.22. Cuban sandwich Quesadilla
Ingredients:
2 slices of reduced fat Swiss (preferably Sargento)
12 inch of low carb whole-wheat tortilla (preferably, La Tortilla Factory)
4 oz. of skinny slow cooked pernil
2 oz. ham (preferably, Hillshire Farm 97% fat free)
2 slices of kosher pickle
Mustard
Directions:
First, you heat a non-stick pan over low heat.
After which you spray with cooking spray and place tortilla on pan.
After that, you place a piece of cheese, pork, ham, pickle and mustard on half of the tortilla.
At a point when cheese melts, you then fold the quesadilla in half and flip to heat other side.
Finally, you remove from heat and cut into 3 pieces
Nutritional value:
Amount per serving: 1 serving size
Calories: 185.8
Fat: 8.7g
Carbohydrate: 23.2g
Dietary fiber: 7.2g
Protein: 23.2g

3.23. Chicken and Andouille Sausage

Ingredients:
2 cups of chopped onion
½ cup of chopped celery
24 oz. of lean skinless chicken drumsticks, with bon
2 teaspoons of all-purpose flour (preferably, rice flour for gluten-free)
4 links (12 oz.) Andouille chicken/turkey sausage (Applegate)
½ cup of chopped scallion
4 teaspoons of oil
1 cup of chopped green bell pepper
28 oz. of lean skinless chicken thighs, with bone
Salt and fresh pepper
4 cups of water
2 bay leaves

Directions:
1. First, you heat a large deep non-stick skillet over medium heat.

2. At a point when it is hot, you add the oil, onions, peppers and celery.

3. After which you cook for about 3 to 4 minutes, stirring.

4. After that, you push the vegetables to the edges of the skillet and add the chicken, season with salt and pepper.

5. Brown for about 2 to 3 minutes on each side, then sprinkle the flour over the chicken and vegetables.

6. This is when you add the water, sausage and bay leaf, adjust salt and pepper to taste, then cover and reduce heat to low.

7. Then you simmer for about 30 to 35 minutes, remove bay leaf and top with scallions.

8. When serve, I suggest you with rice or quinoa if desired.

Nutritional value:
Amount per serving: 1 serving size
Calories: 347.5
Fat: 13g
Carbohydrate: 8g
Dietary fiber: 2g
Protein: 47g

3.24. CONCLUSION

These healthy recipes would help you Shred the Fat Instantly and keep the weight off for good. Get in shape this Season taking this Delectable Recipes. If you follow religiously to the #Eat. Nourish. Glow.: 10 easy steps for losing weight, looking younger & feeling healthier By Amelia Freer and some of the recipes outlined in this book. You are going to be seeing results in 14days, because it is proven to work.

3.24.1. Thank You

However, if you enjoyed the recipes in this book, please take the time to share your thoughts and post a positive review with 5 star rating on Amazon, it would make me serve you better. It'd be greatly appreciated!
Thank you and good luck!

CPSIA information can be obtained at www.ICGtesting.com
Printed in the USA
LVOW04s0520040515

437112LV00028B/925/P

9 781511 403566